OLIVER the BRAVE ©

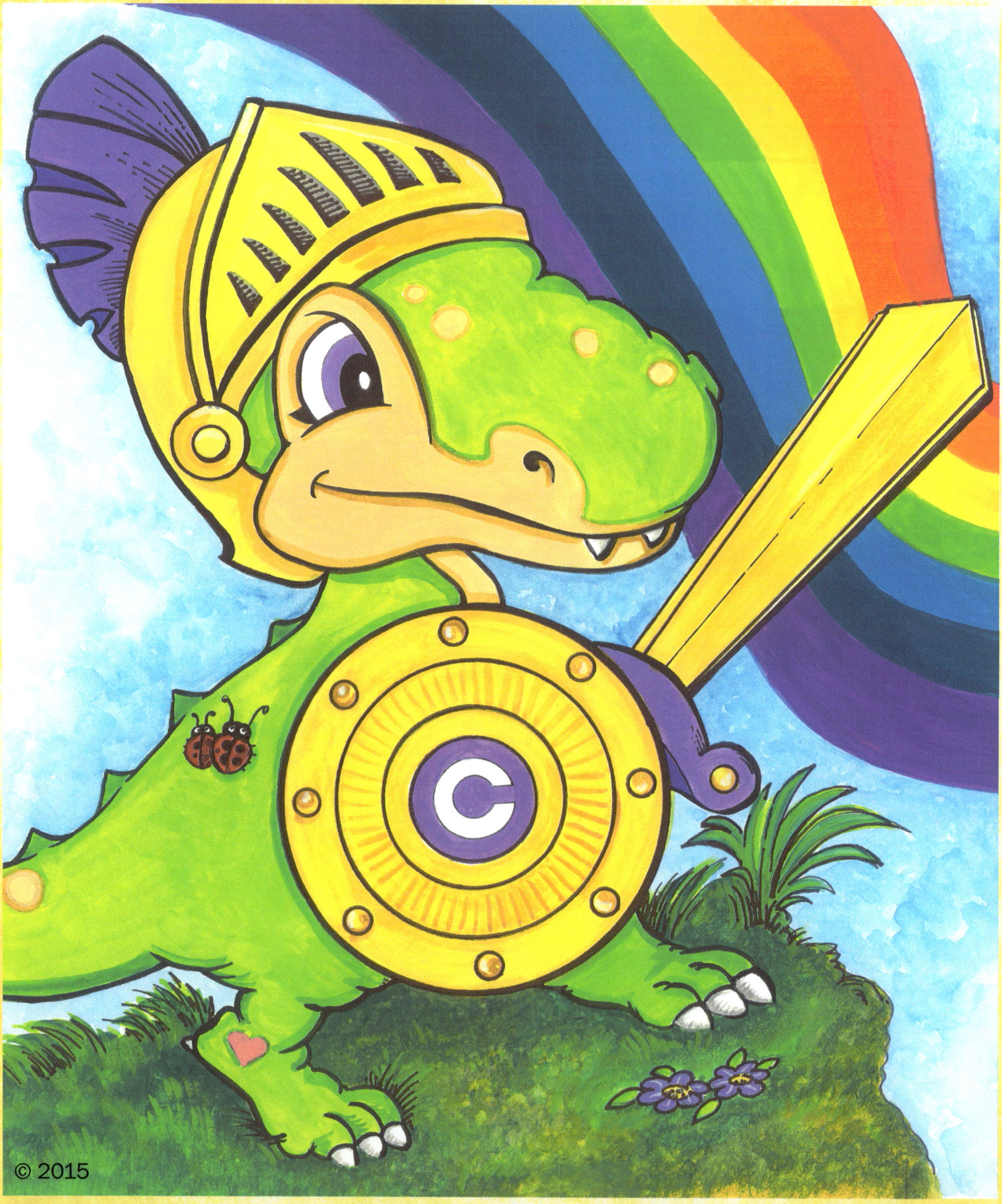
© 2015

OLIVER the BRAVE©

DEFENDER of CHILDREN, DESTROYER of CANCER

Fighting Childhood Cancer

Written and illustrated by
Lynn Faherty

Graphic Designer
Patricia Paisley

For more information visit us at:
www.oliverthebrave.com

This book is dedicated to
CARSYN VOLPE
The brave and strong warrior
who inspired this story.
I say,
"You are Brave, You are Strong,
I Believe it!"
LF

I hope that this story will help you and your family during your battle with cancer. Always remember that you are not alone.
You are a lifetime member of
The Order of the Golden Sword and Shield!
You are a brave and courageous warrior just like me!
NEVER GIVE UP!

Just say,

"I am Brave, I am Strong, I BELIEVE IT!"

Love,
Oliver

This Book Belongs To:

BRAVE WARRIOR,

____

A proud member of the
Order of the Golden Sword and Shield.
A Defender of Children,
A Destroyer of Cancer.
You are Brave, You are Strong,
BELIEVE IT!

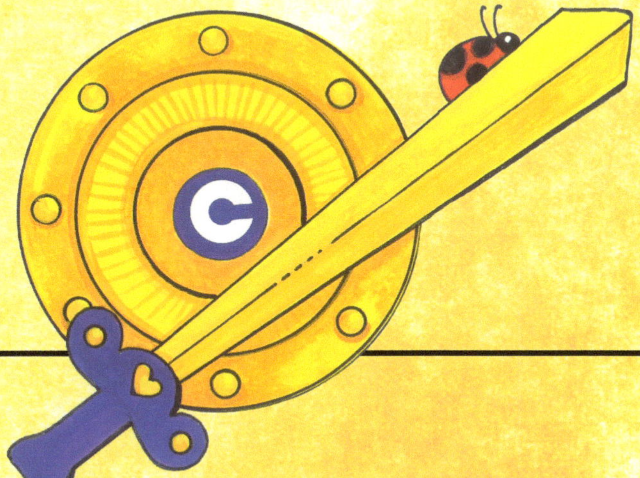

My name is Oliver.
I am a T-Rex.

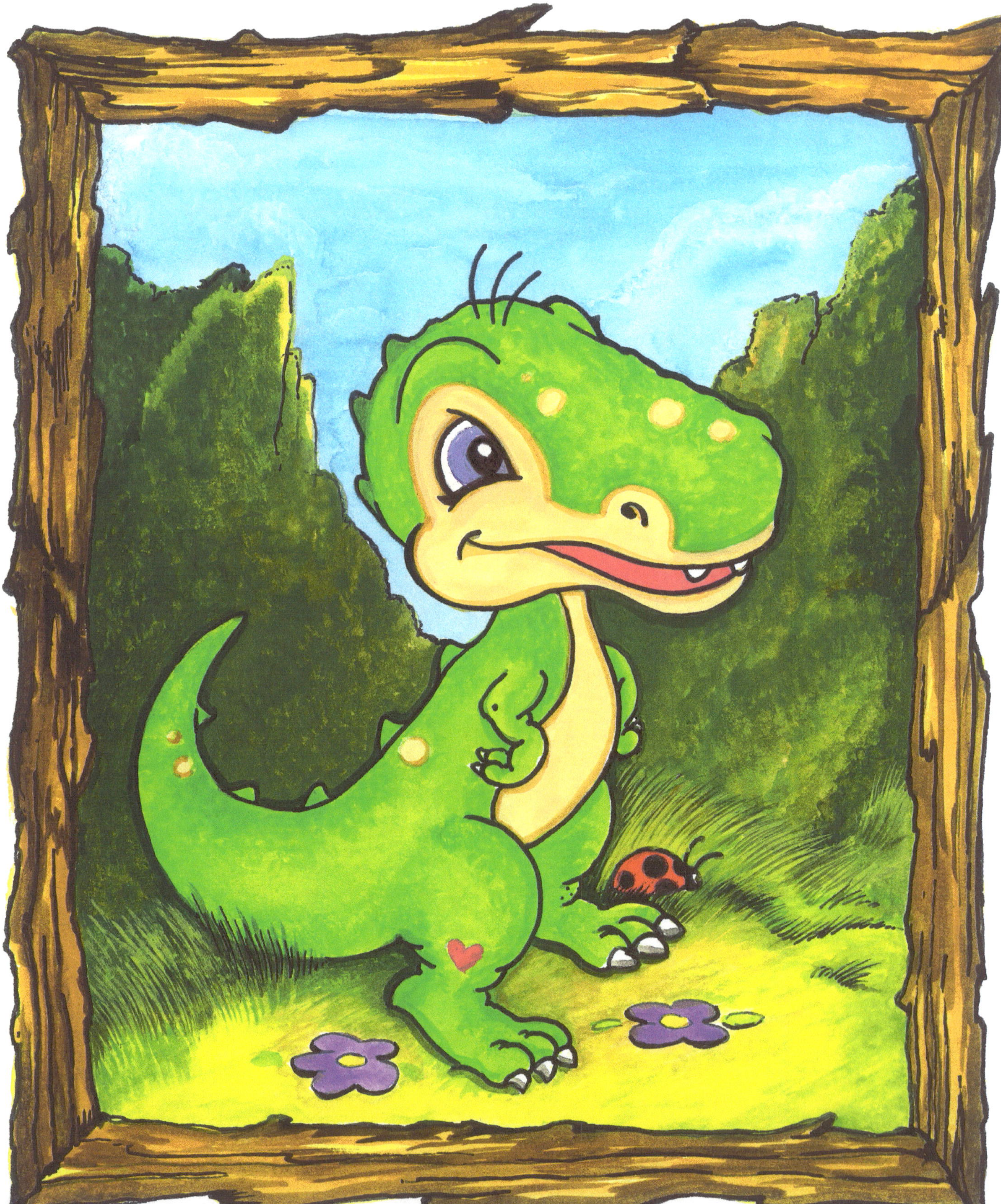

I belong to the mightiest dinosaur family to ever roam the forest. I live with my sisters Opal and Olivia, and our Mom and Dad.

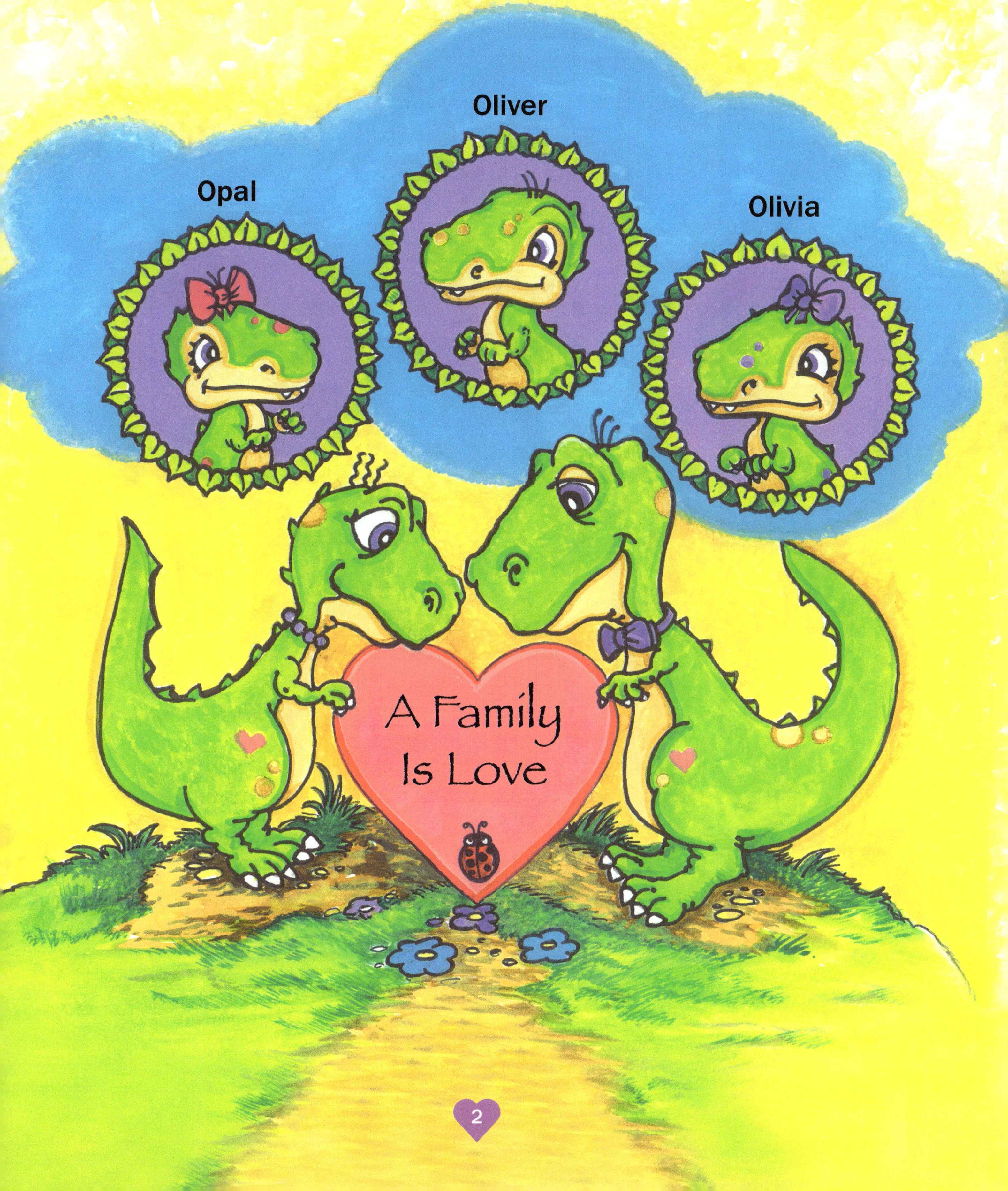

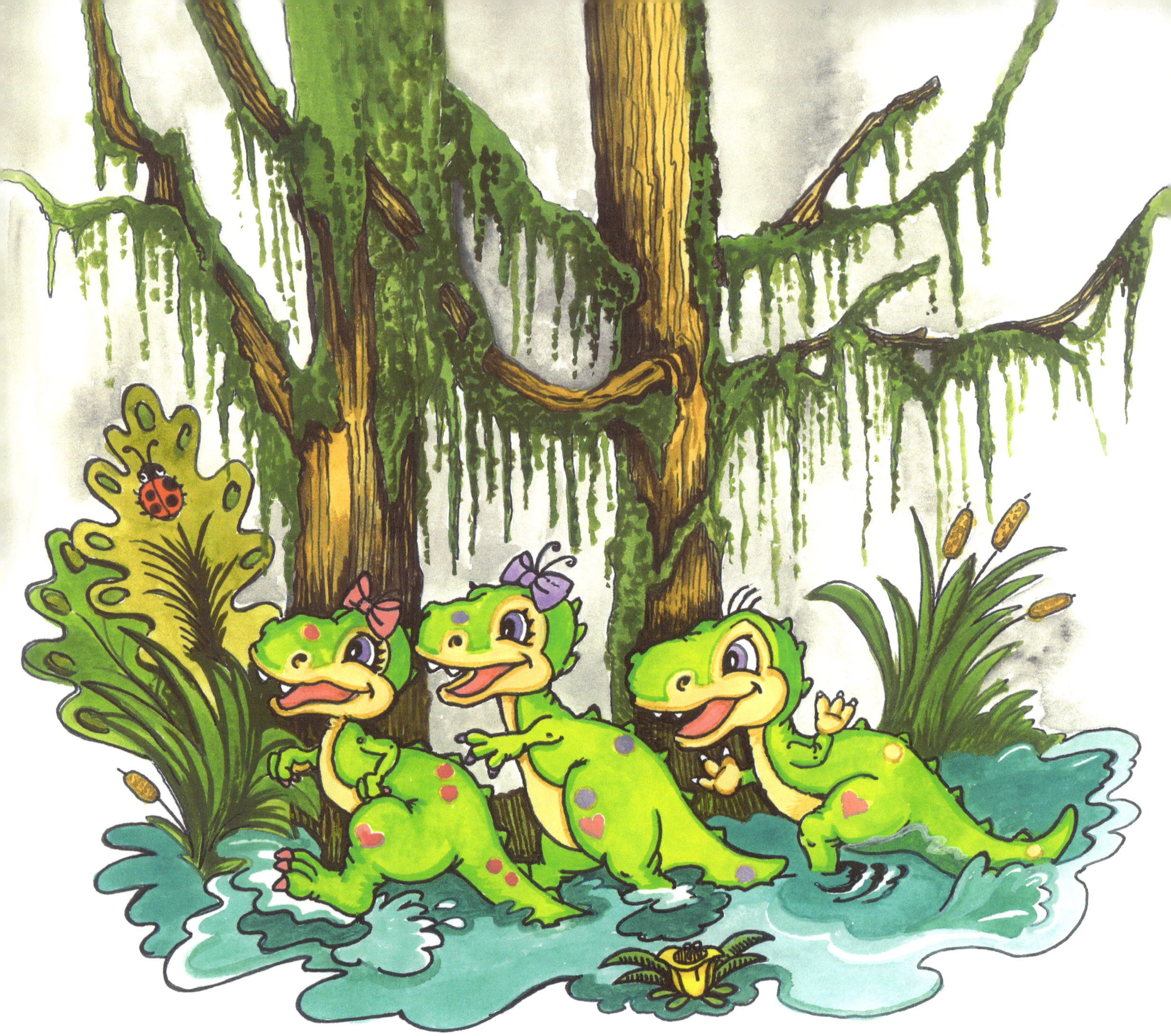

I like to run and play in the forest
and splash through the swamps with my sisters.

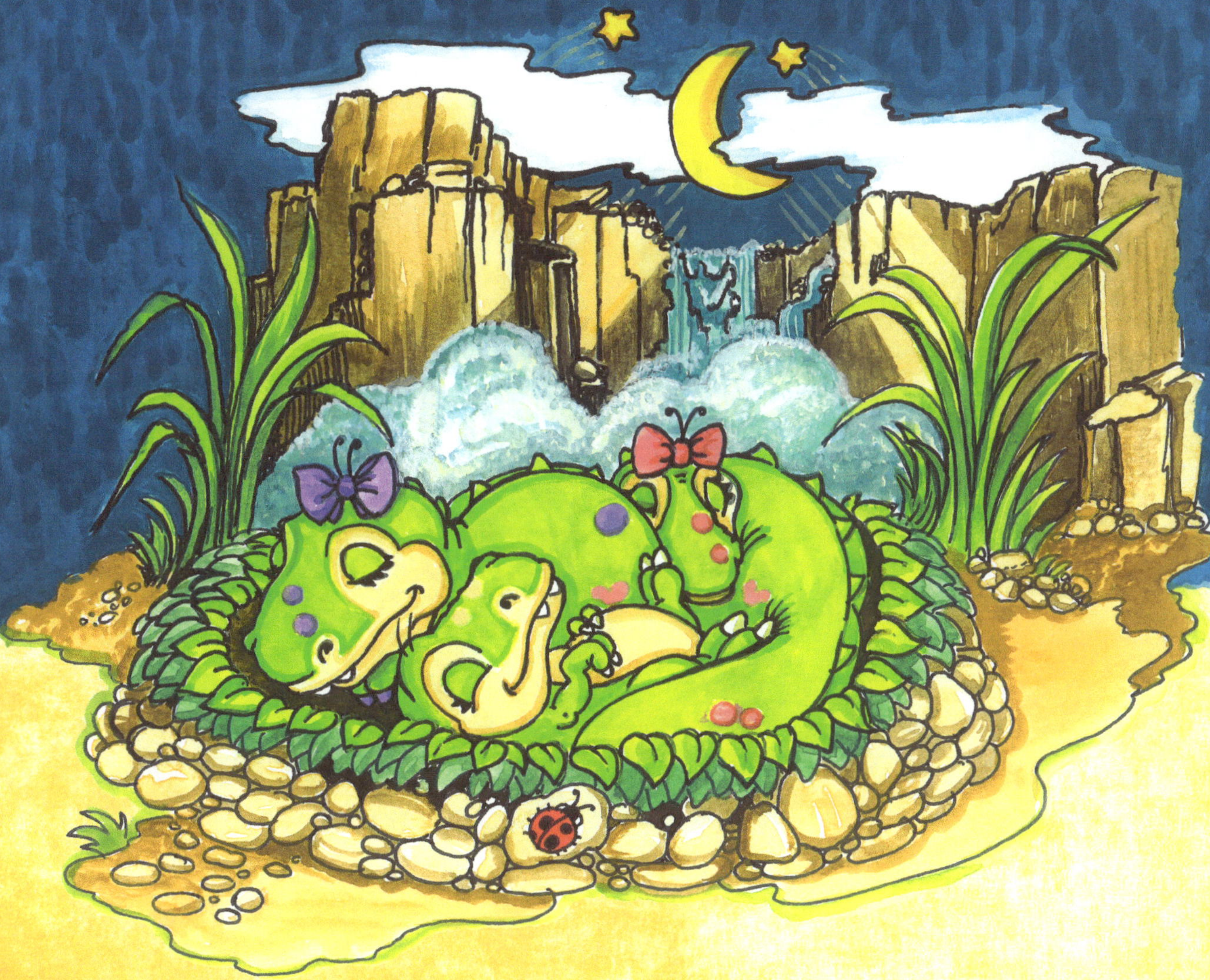

Life in the forest was good. Nothing ever seemed to change.
Eat, play, sleep. It was always the same.
At night we slept in our nest.
It's the place we called home where we always felt safe.

Suddenly, I was not myself at all.
I slept a lot and kept getting fevers. I had pain all over my body.
Mom and Dad took me to the doctor. The symptoms I had could have been caused by a virus. We hoped it would just go away.
Mom and Dad took me home.
I didn't feel well. I was frightened.

But I said,

"I am Brave, I am Strong, I BELIEVE IT!"

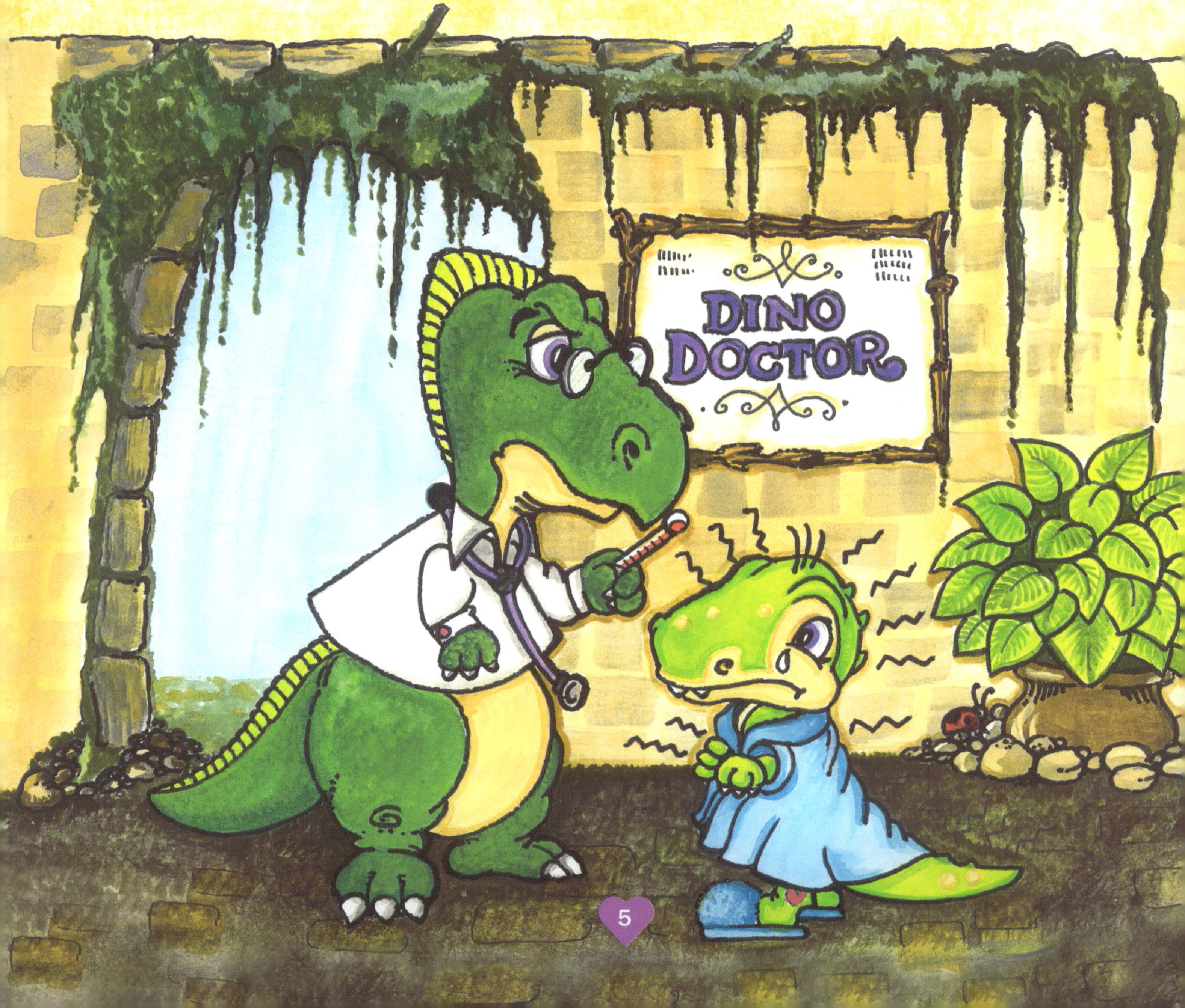

One morning I woke up late and went looking for Opal and Olivia.
I found them having breakfast with Mom.
Right away I could tell something was wrong.
Mom showed me that I had purple rings around my eyes.
I kind of looked like a raccoon. *This,* was not a virus!
I got scared.

But I said,

"I am Brave, I am Strong, I BELIEVE IT!"

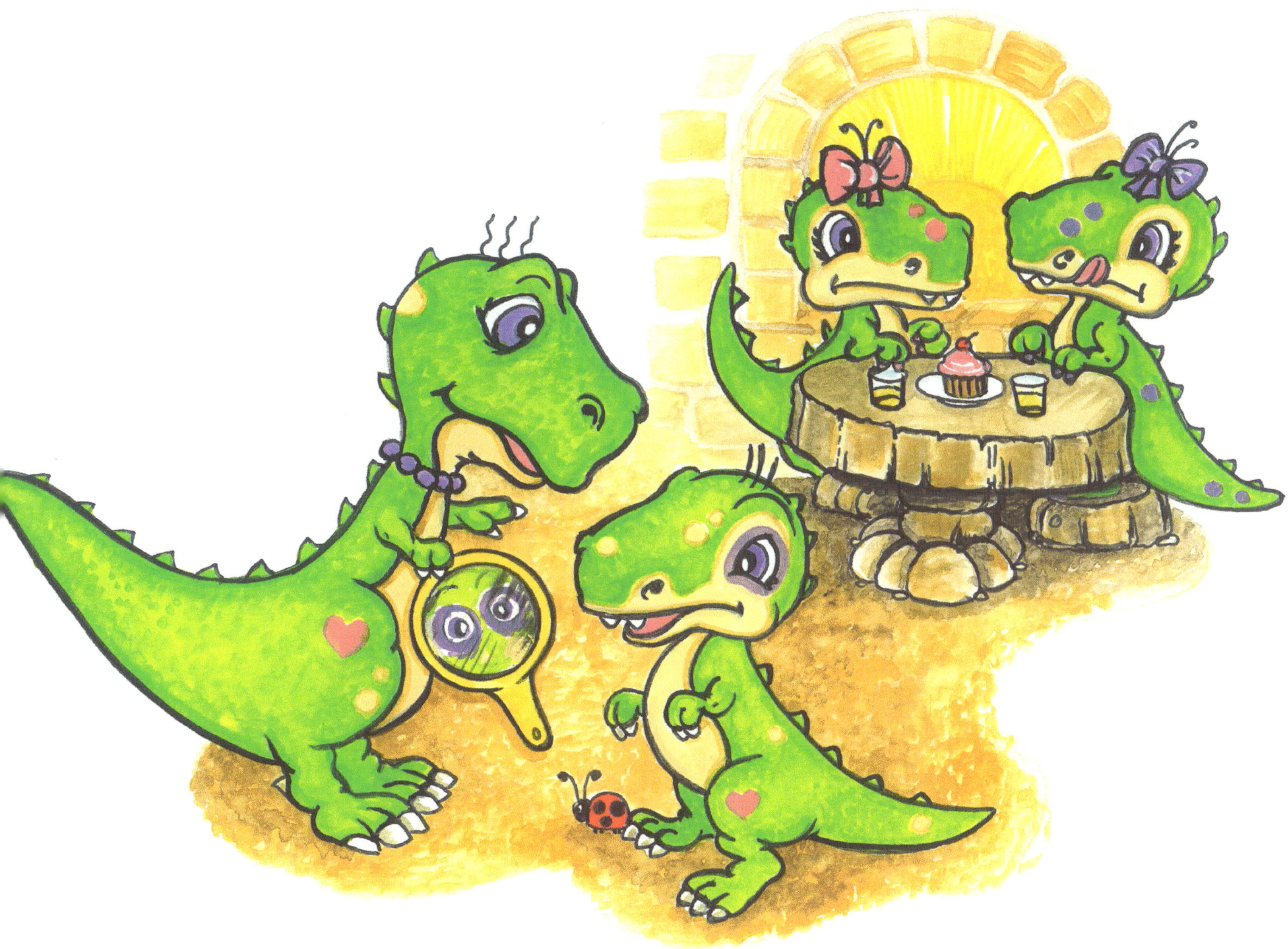

Mom called the doctor.
The doctor said we should go to the hospital.
The hospital was like a big doctors office
with lots of rooms and people rushing in and out.
I had an exam.
Along with the purple rings around my eyes,
the doctor found a lump on my body. He gave me lots of
different tests. All of these tests would DIAGNOSE my illness,
or tell the doctor what was making me feel sick.
I was feeling confused.

When all of the tests were finished,
the doctor told us that I had cancer. Mom was crying.
Dad just hugged me. My sisters were very quiet.
I didn't understand what was going to happen to me.
We met with a very special doctor called an ONCOLOGIST.
He helps people with cancer get better. He said there were ways
that my whole family could get involved too.
We all had lots of questions.

But I said,

"I am Brave, I am Strong, I BELIEVE IT!"

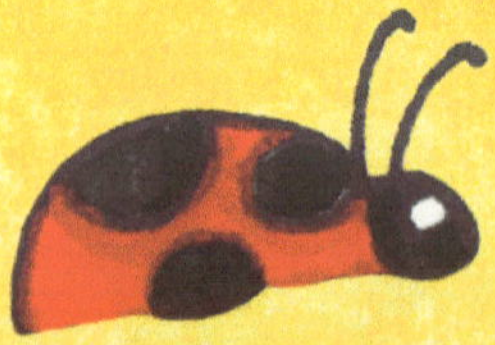

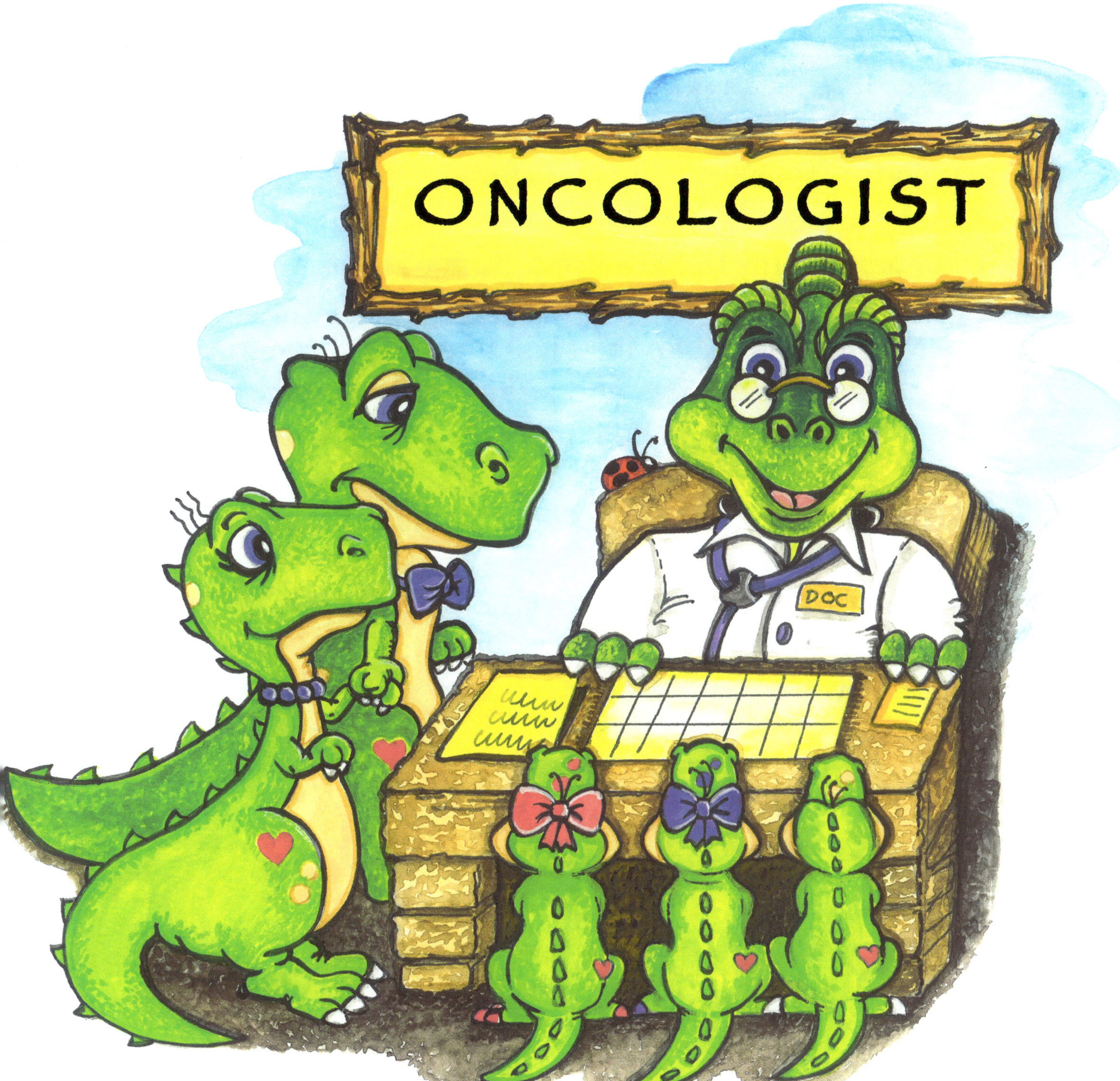
ONCOLOGIST
DOC

I asked the doctor, “What is cancer?”
He explained that cancer is when the cells in one part of your body start to grow out of control and can spread to other parts of your body and make you sick. I asked him if it was my fault that I got cancer. I wondered if my family or friends could catch it from me. He told me that I did nothing wrong, no one can catch cancer. No one was to blame, it just happens sometimes. I got lots of hugs and kisses from my family. I was feeling really sad.

He said that children from different places around the world have cancer too. There are many kinds of cancer. I was glad to know that I wasn’t alone, and there are special medicines to make me feel better. Doctors and scientists are working on new treatments everyday! We hope and pray for a cure! We don’t know why I got cancer.

But I said,

“I am Brave, I am Strong, I BELIEVE IT!”

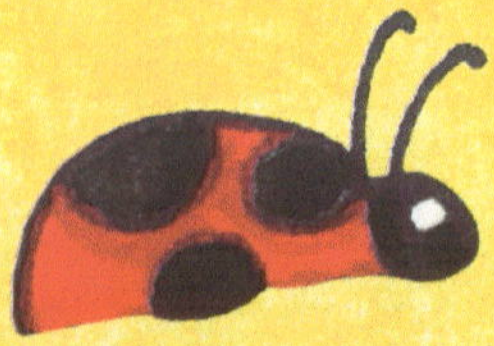

WE NEED A

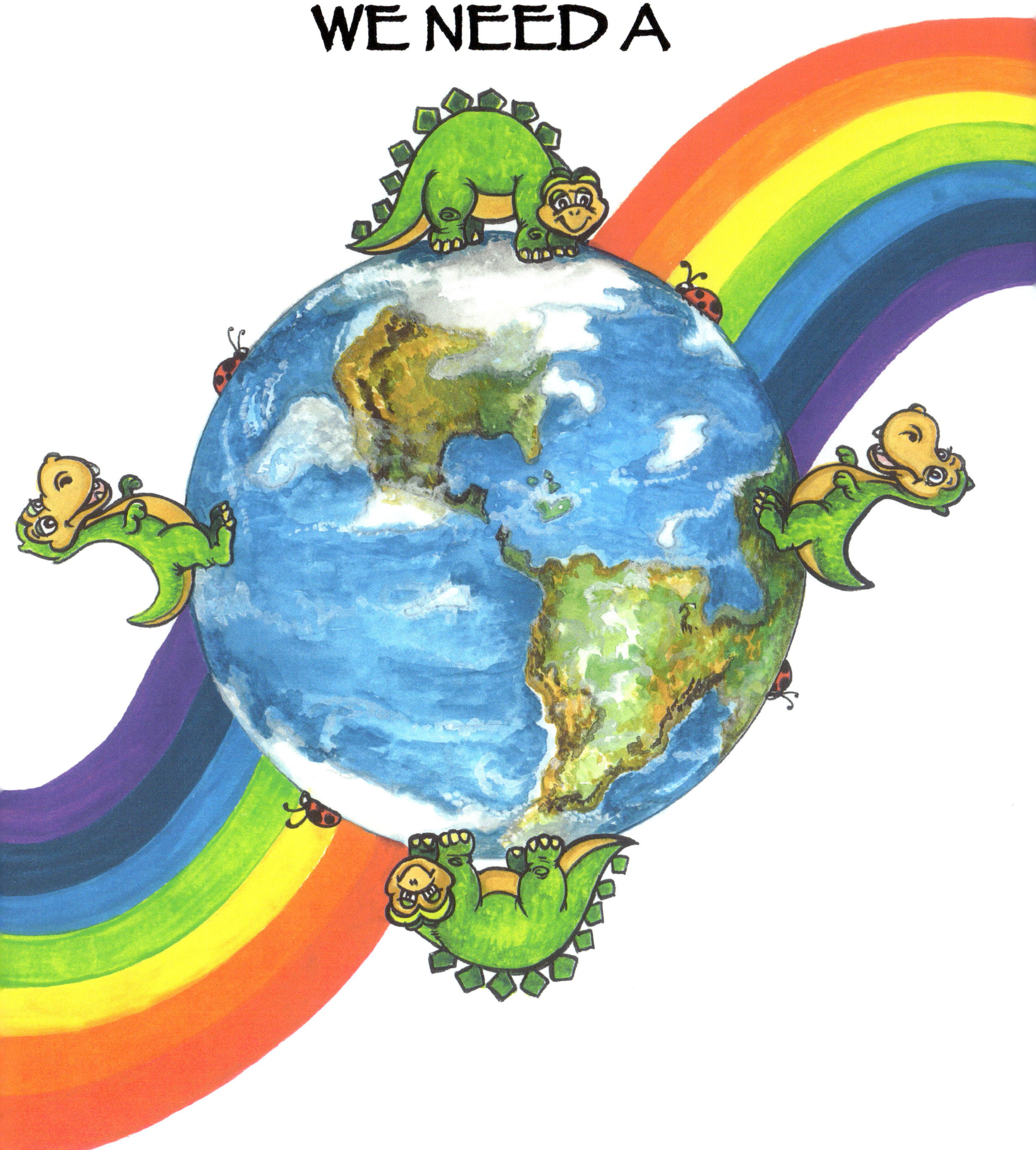

CANCER-FREE WORLD!

The doctor explained that I would need a very strong medicine called CHEMOTHERAPY. This medicine would destroy the bad cancer cells in my body. I had to be in the hospital to get this treatment. He said it was very important to start right away. My nurse gave me the CHEMOTHERAPY through a PORT, which is a special passage she put into my body.

I also had a treatment called RADIATION THERAPY. It's given by a machine that uses high-energy x-rays to shrink tumors and destroy cancer cells. I couldn't feel it or smell it, I just had to lay still. This treatment didn't take too long. My team of doctors and nurses have very important jobs. They were really nice and funny too. They always explained what they were going to do to me and how it might feel. They helped me make a treatment journal.
We became friends.
Now I felt brave, instead of afraid!

So I said,
"I am Brave, I am Strong, I BELIEVE IT!"

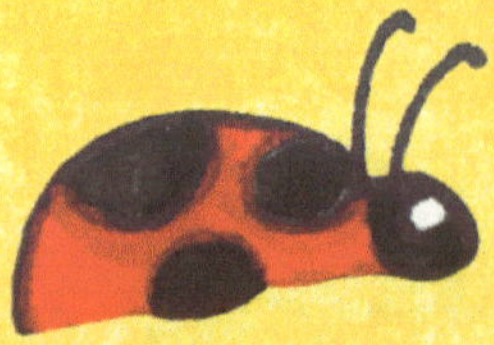

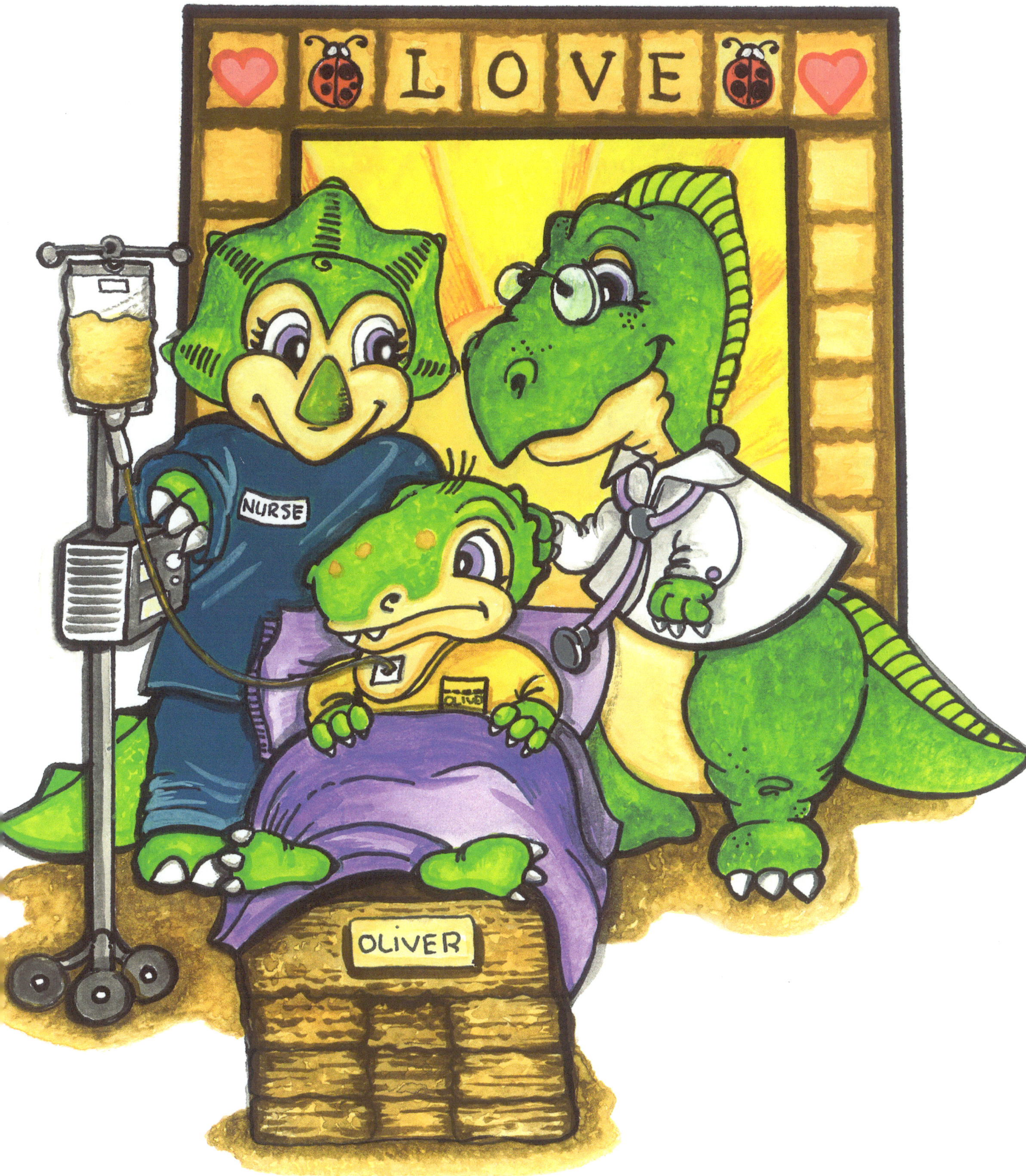
LOVE
NURSE
OLIVER

CHEMOTHERAPY was hard.
I got very sick.
I threw up.
I got very weak.
I even lost my hair!

Mom explained it would grow back.
She said I could wear wigs, scarves, or hats,
whatever made me feel good.
My Dad surprised me when he shaved off
his own hair.
We were bald buddies.

So I said,
"I am Brave, I am Strong, I BELIEVE IT!"

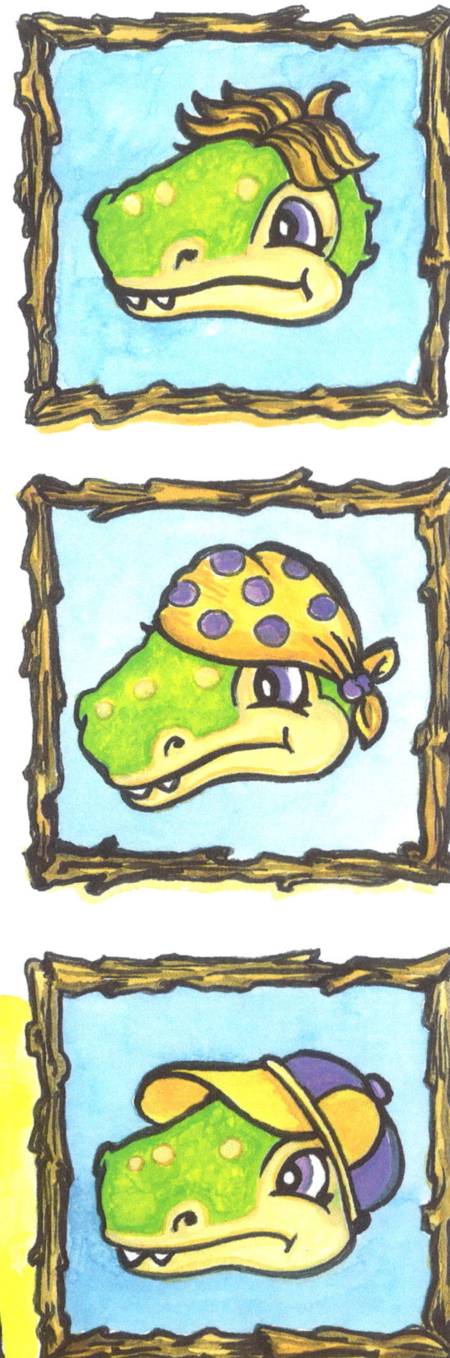

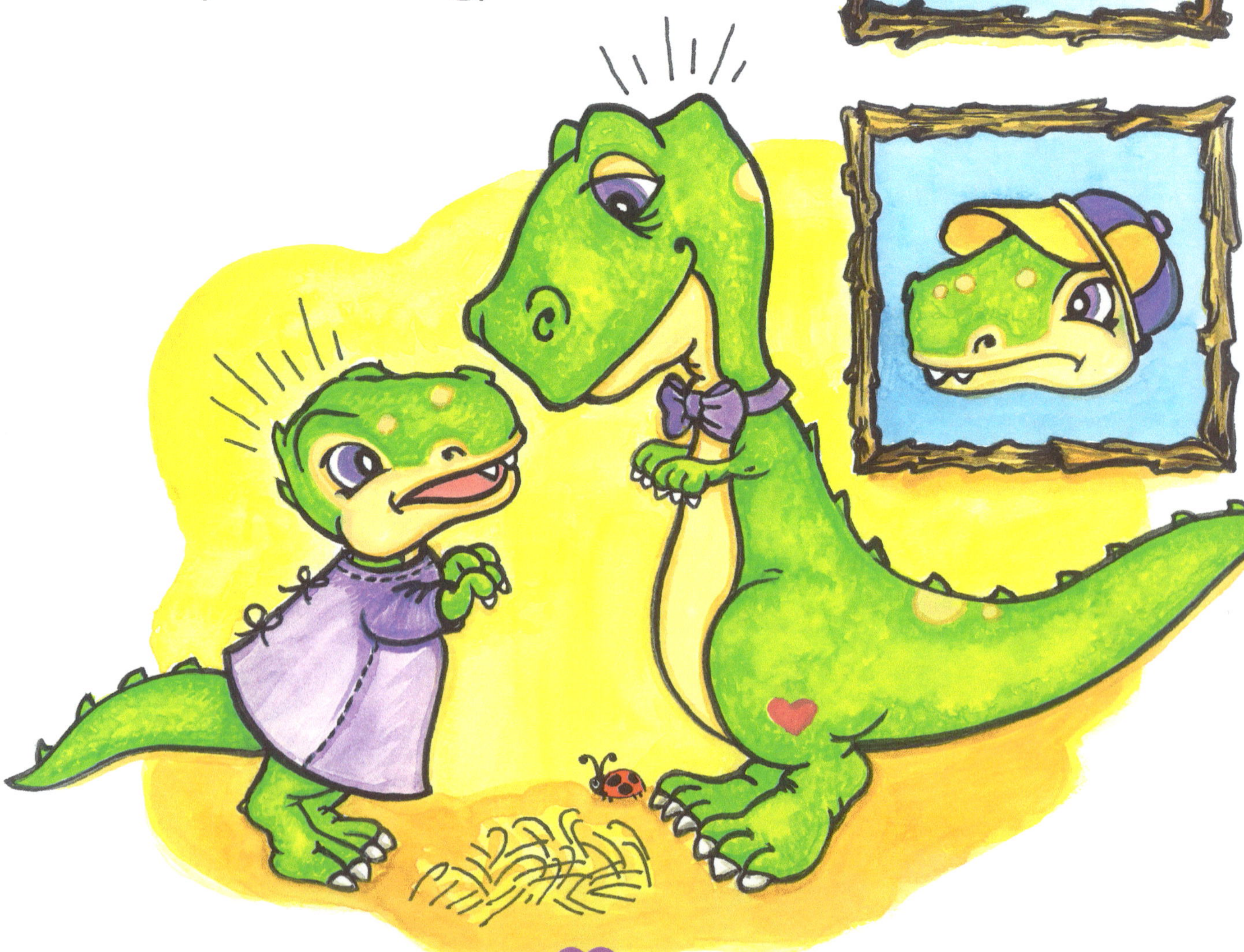

While I was in the hospital, my family spent lots of time with me. Every day was all about me. Sometimes I felt bad for my sisters. They couldn't get all of the attention that they deserved while Mom and Dad were caring for me. I was given so many nice cards and gifts. Many people prayed for me. Mom and Dad never stopped telling me how much they loved me. Everyone was so proud of me for being such a fighter. They said I was their brave warrior! I fought really hard to get better.

So I said,

"I am Brave, I am Strong, I BELIEVE IT!"

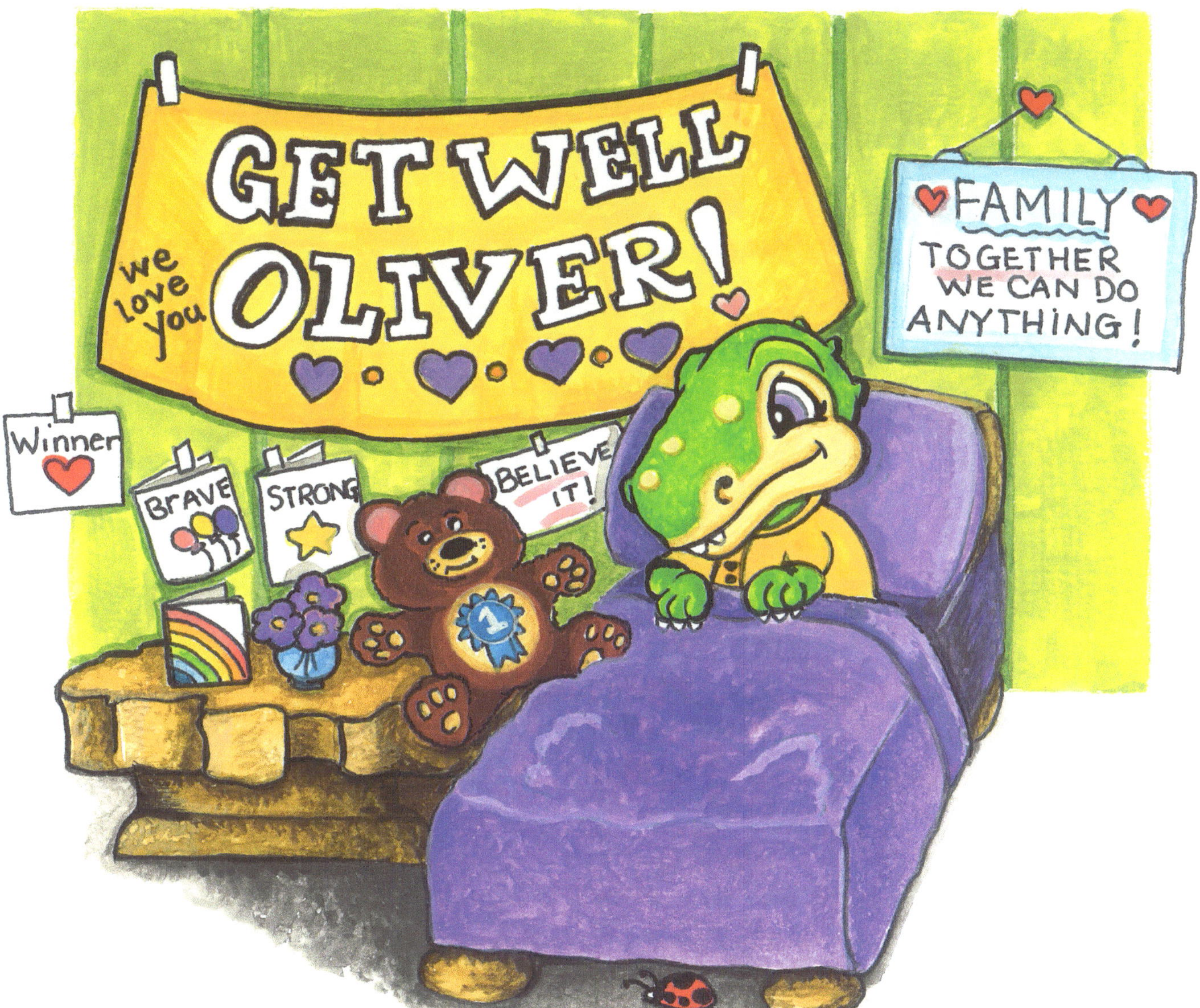
GET WELL OLIVER!
we love you
FAMILY
TOGETHER WE CAN DO ANYTHING!
Winner
Brave
STRONG
BELIEVE IT!
1

I learned that every cancer is different. Every patient gets a special treatment plan. I was given a test on my BONE MARROW, the stuff inside my bones that makes my blood cells. My doctors thought it would be a good idea to save my STEM CELLS. These cells grow into the three types of cells that make up my blood. They took out my STEM CELLS and saved them until all of the cancer cells in my body had been destroyed. I had to have more CHEMOTHERAPY. I got very weak. My family cheered me on! I knew they were worried.

But I said,

"I am Brave, I am Strong, I BELIEVE IT!"

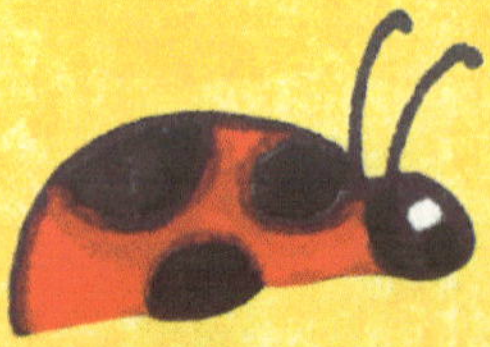

My sisters were amazing! When I felt sad, Opal and Olivia did funny things to make me laugh. They became "Team Oliver." My family gave me strength and hope. They made me fight to get better. When the cancer cells were gone, my doctors put my STEM CELLS back inside my bones so they could grow lots of healthy new cells. The new cells took time to start growing. We waited and waited and waited. It seemed like forever!

But I said,

"I am Brave, I am Strong, I BELIEVE IT!"

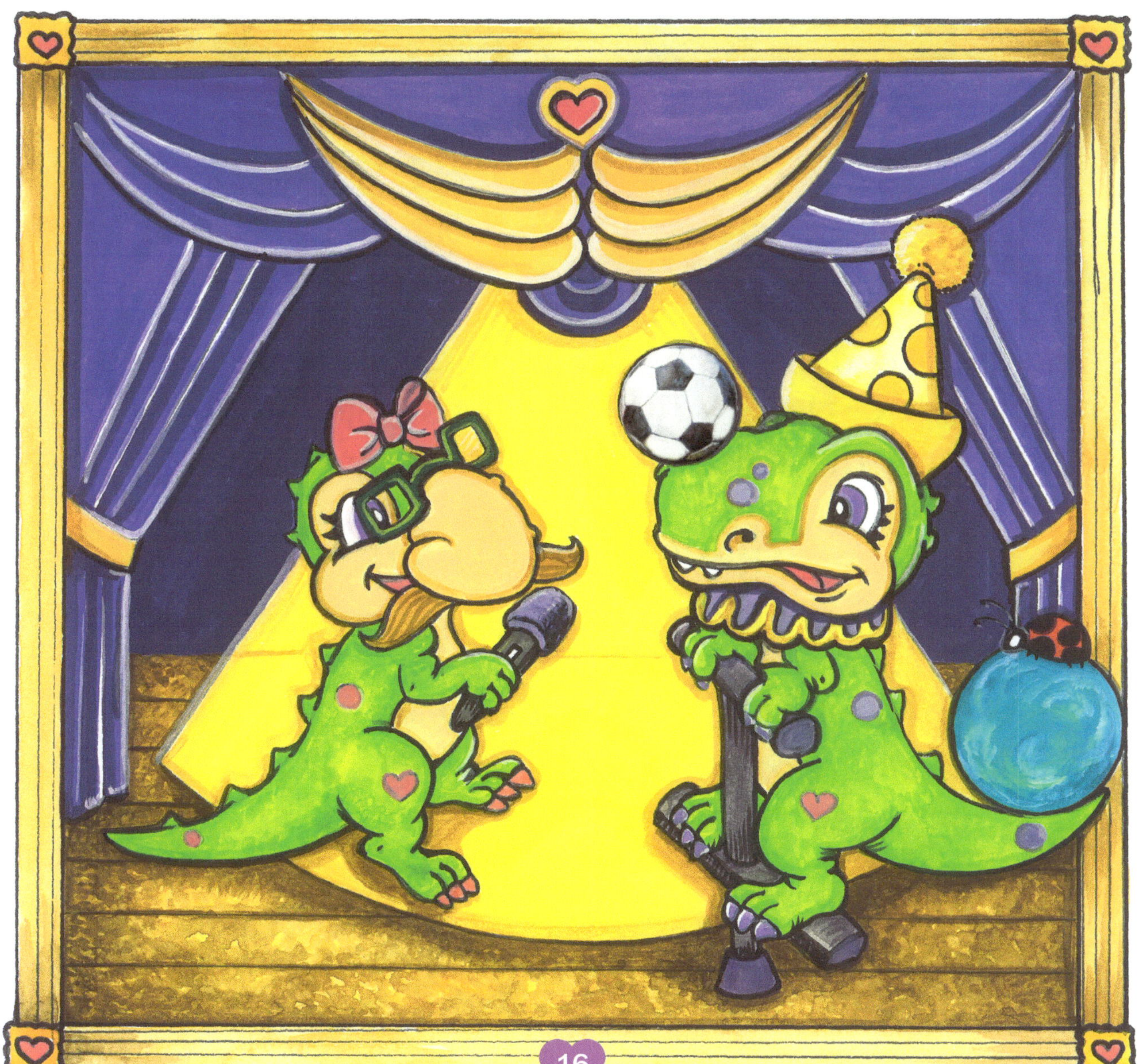

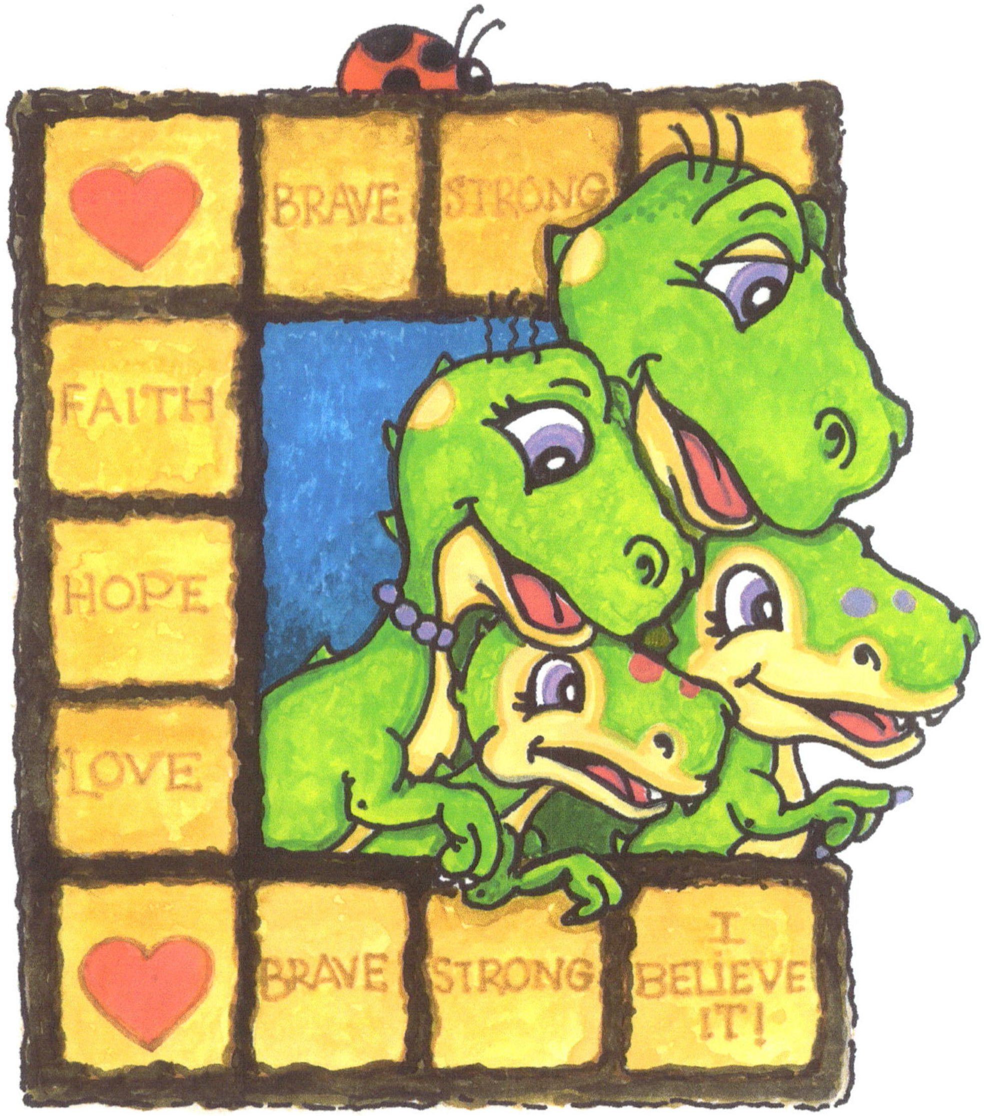

We grew tired of waiting. Finally the cells began to grow!
A huge CELL-EBRATION! This was called REBIRTH!
This was the moment I became...

OLIVER THE BRAVE
Defender of Children, Destroyer of Cancer!

I could feel the super powers growing inside my body
with a strong colorful energy as bright as a rainbow!
I now had the strength to continue this battle.

So I said,
"I am Brave, I am Strong, I BELIEVE IT!"

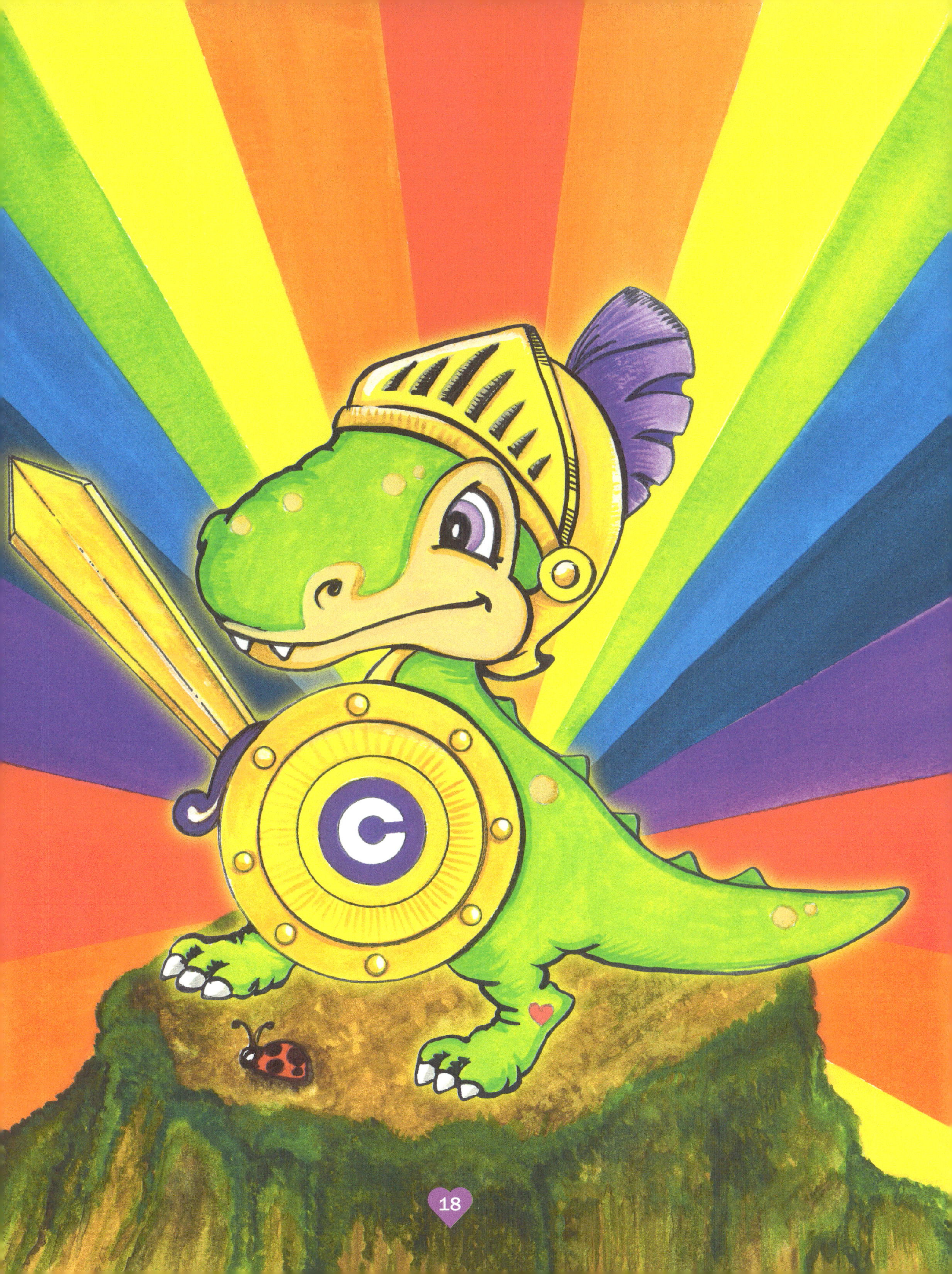
C

I heard a voice inside me saying,
"Oliver, you are brave, you are strong, you must believe it!
Don't ever quit!
KEEP FIGHTING!"

My family could see me changing.
Their little Oliver had become an unstoppable, courageous, warrior!
Their love had created a golden sword and shield to protect me.
I grew stronger each day.
I was no longer afraid.
I felt powerful!

So I said,
"I am Brave, I am Strong, I BELIEVE IT!"

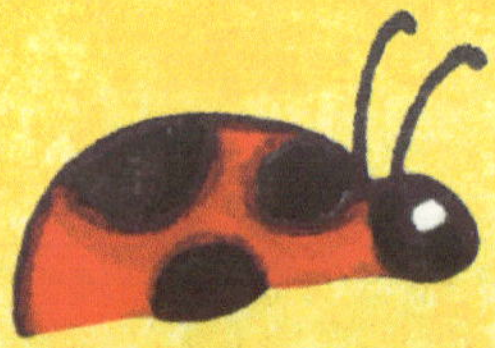

Armed with my golden sword and shield, I turned all of my strength and energy towards healing my body. The CHEMOTHERAPY had destroyed my body's good blood cells along with the bad cancer cells. All of my germ-fighting blood cells were gone. I could get very sick, even if I caught a cold.

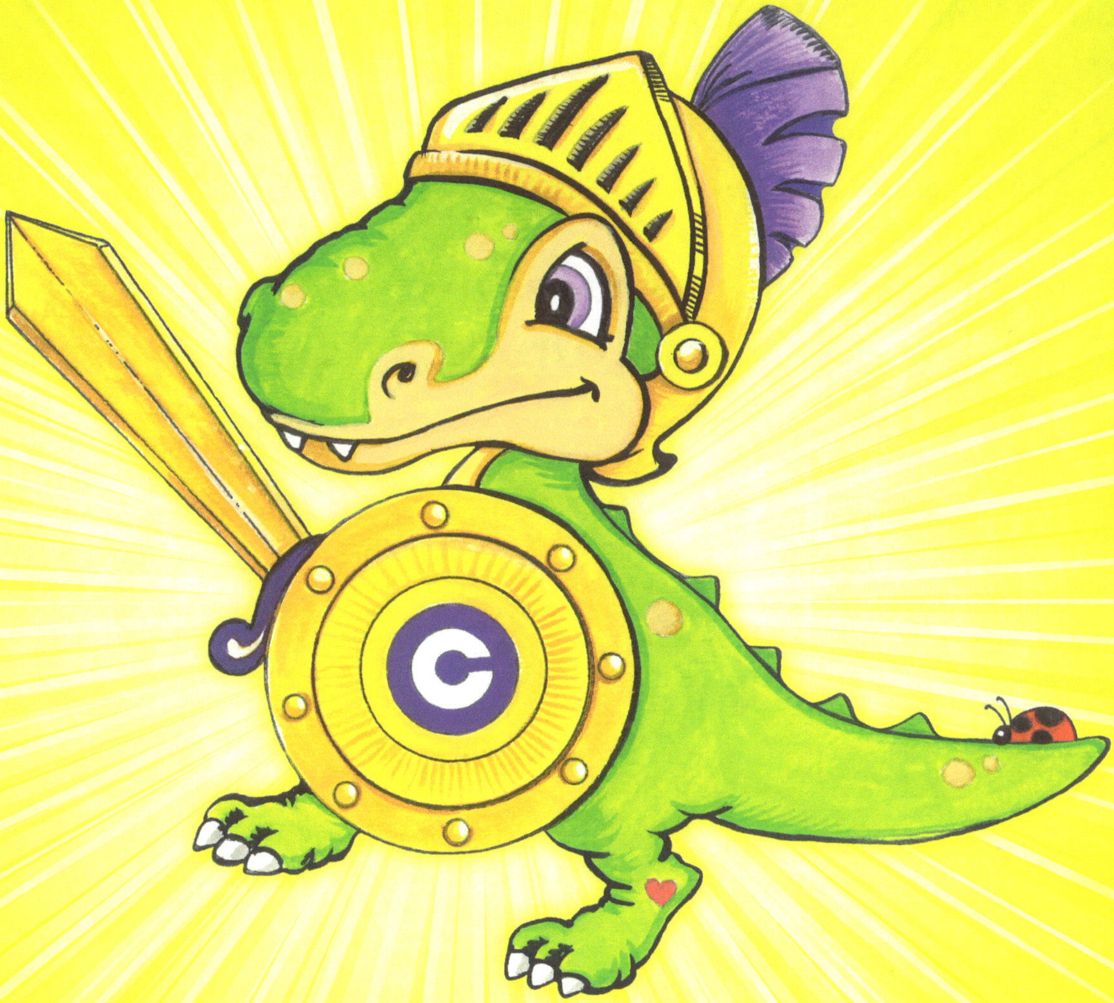

To keep me healthy, I began a treatment called IMMUNOTHERAPY. Together with special medicine, this therapy would help my body find the cancer cells and destroy them. This treatment was followed by a series of shots. I don't really like shots.

But I said,

"I am Brave, I am Strong, I BELIEVE IT!"

We had to make sure that our home stayed germ free. It was important that Opal and Olivia stayed healthy too. Sometimes we had to miss school. I had to stay away from crowds and wear a mask. We had many late night trips to the hospital. Fighting cancer was hard on our whole family. There were times when we got angry with each other. We were tired and feeling kind of stressed. It was hard to follow so many rules. Mom and Dad taught me to eat healthy and rest, so my body would continue to heal. Over time we could see that all of the hard work was worth it. My treatment was finished. I was getting better!

And I said,

"I am Brave, I am Strong, I BELIEVE IT!"

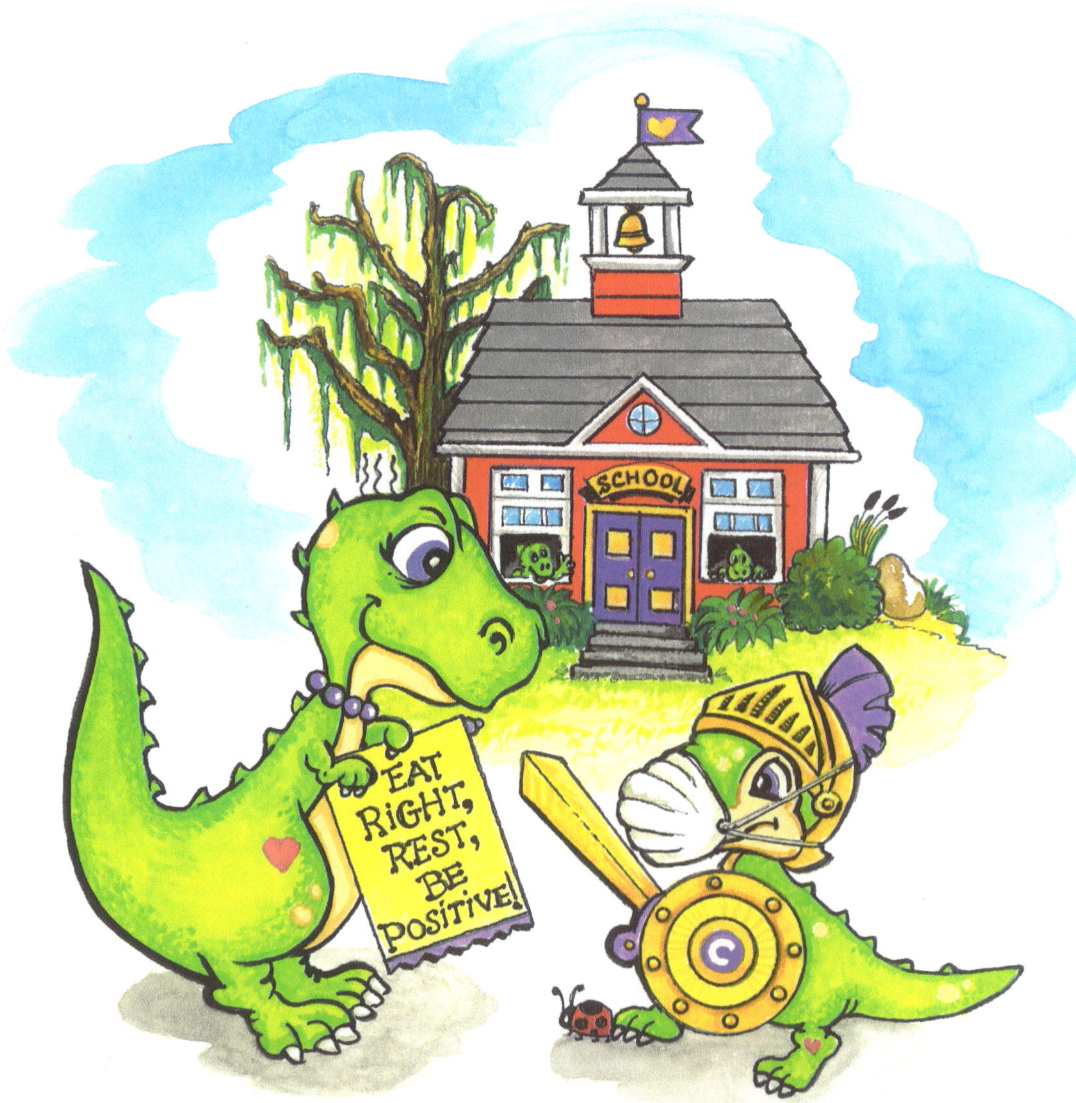

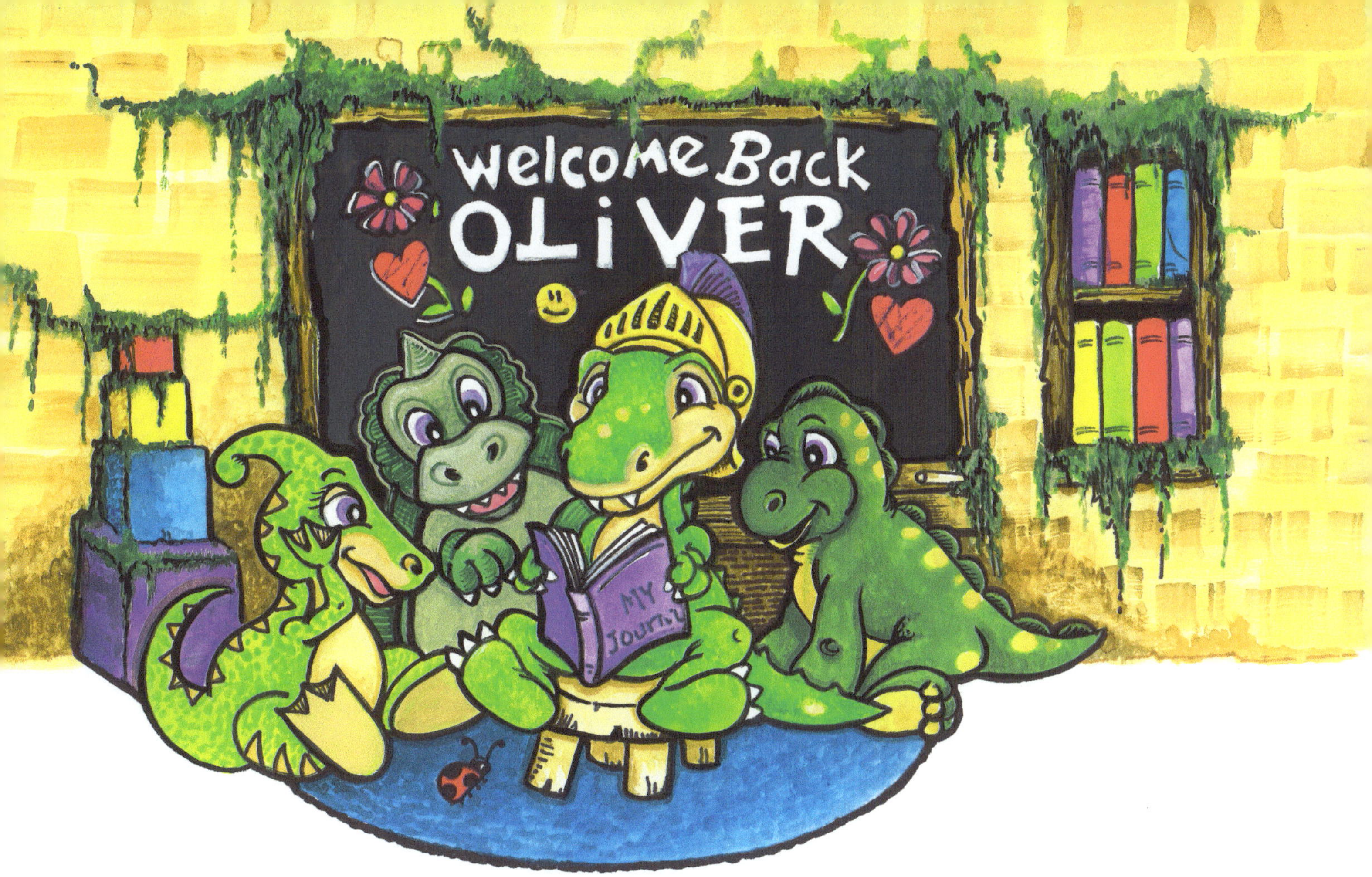

With a good check up, my doctor said I could return to school.
I felt kind of nervous. My hair was still growing back.
My teacher helped me tell the class that I had cancer.
I didn't want them to be afraid of me. I told them about CHEMOTHERAPY, and why I lost my hair.
I thanked everyone for the cards and gifts they sent to me.
They made me feel so special.
I shared my treatment journal with the class.
Everything was better after my friends learned about cancer.
They knew it was okay to be close to me again.
They believed that Oliver the Brave was a super hero!
They wanted to be on "Team Oliver" too.
That made me really happy!

So I said,

"I am Brave, I am Strong, I BELIEVE IT!"

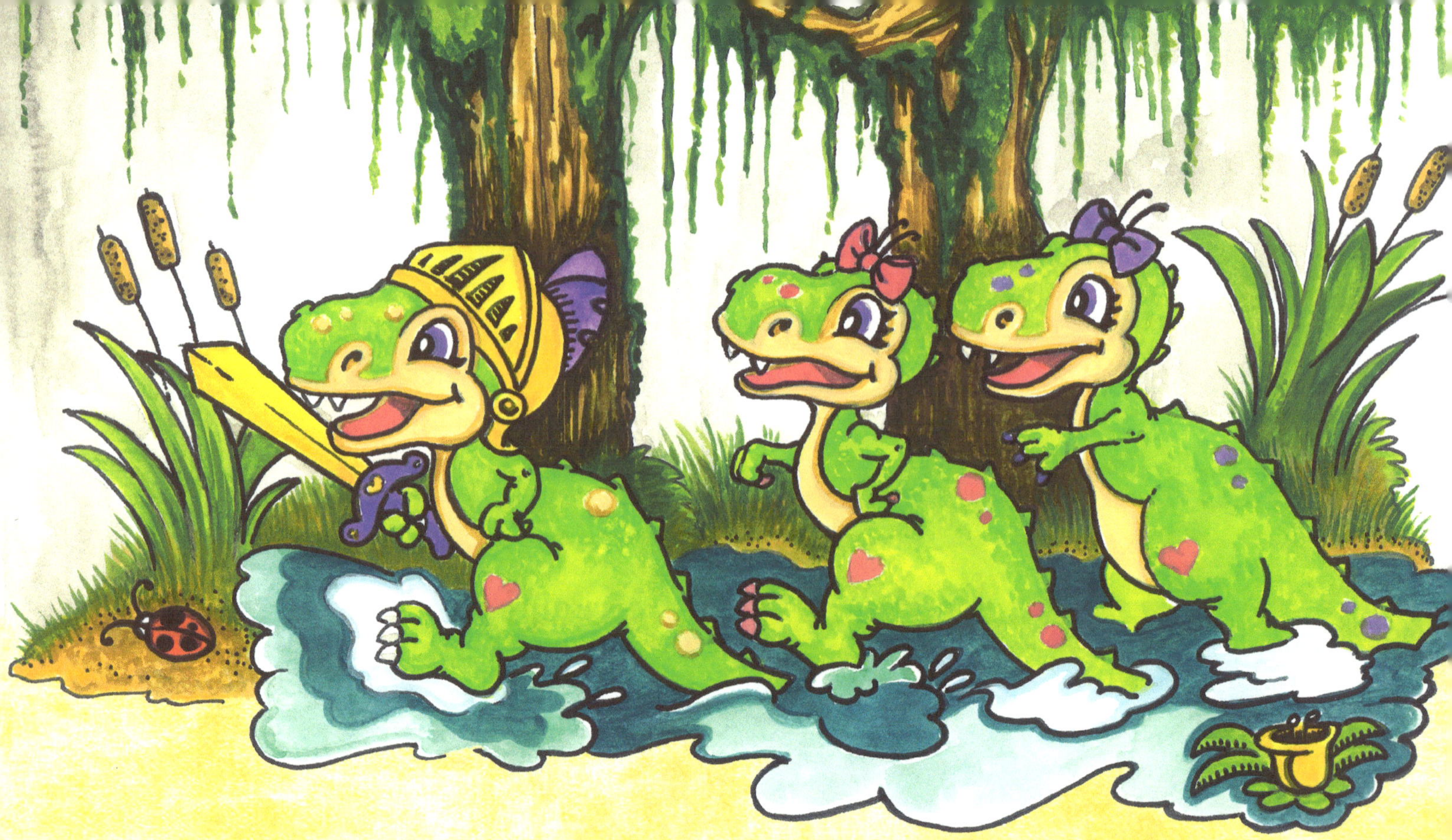

Fighting cancer was hard, but I am strong!
I am back to running and playing in the forest and splashing through the swamps with my sisters. I still have to go for check-ups to make sure the cancer cells have not come back. It's okay because everyday is a miracle. I am so grateful to be able to share my journey with you and your family. I can still remember when I first got cancer. I felt so afraid. There are times when I still get scared.
Then I hear a voice deep inside my heart,
and it whispers at first...

"I am Brave, I am Strong, I BELIEVE IT!"

Then it gets a little louder...

"I am Brave, I am Strong, I BELIEVE IT!"

Then I need to shout!

"I am Brave, I am Strong, I BELIEVE IT!"

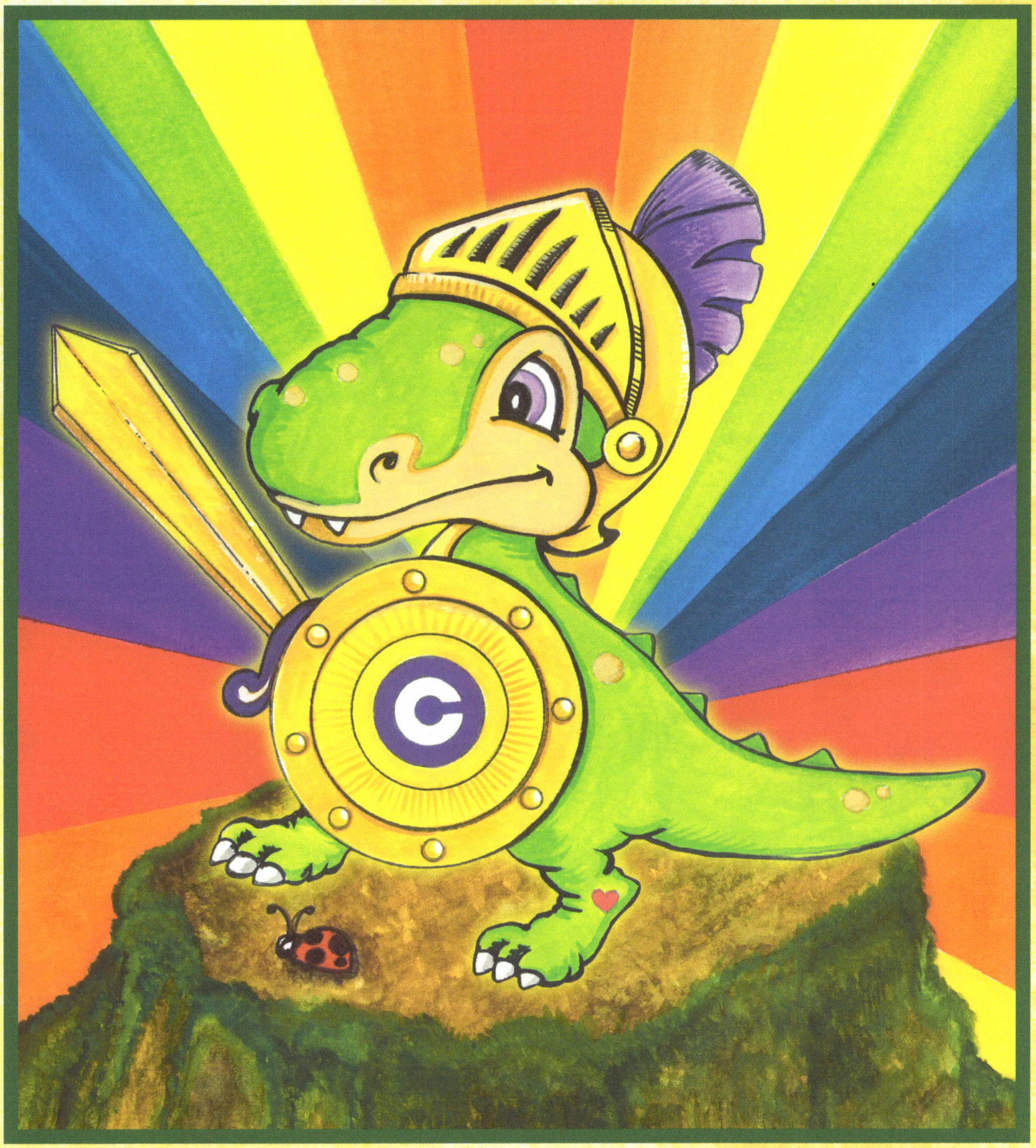

I can feel the super powers growing inside my body again...
Now I know I will always
have the strength for any battle,
and I BELIEVE IT!

www.ingramcontent.com/pod-product-compliance
Lightning Source LLC
LaVergne TN
LVHW070956210926
848482LV00002B/226